VEGETARIAN RECIPES FOR TYPE 1 DIABETICS

Delicious & Balanced Meals for Managing Type 1 Diabetes with Plant-Based Power

T. John

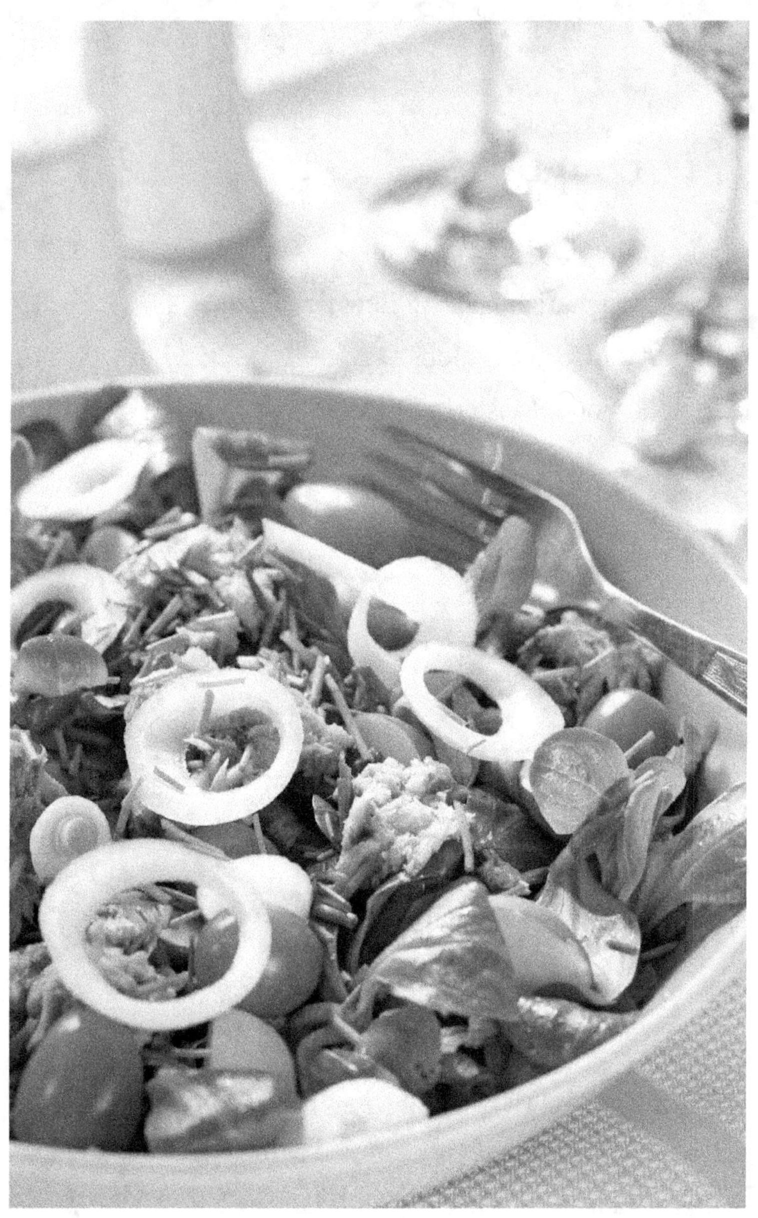

TABLE OF CONTENTS

Chapter 5: Snacks and Appetizers 92

Chapter 6: Desserts 113

INTRODUCTION

I magine your body's incredible ability to use food for energy is disrupted. That's the reality for those living with Type 1 Diabetes, an autoimmune condition where the pancreas stops producing insulin, the key that unlocks cells to absorb glucose (sugar) from the bloodstream. This imbalance throws blood sugar levels into a constant flux, demanding careful management.

Food: The Keystone of Control

While there's no magic bullet, a well-balanced diet becomes a powerful tool. Unlike Type 2 Diabetes, where dietary changes might influence insulin production, the focus here shifts to managing blood sugar response to food. Carbohydrates, the body's primary source of energy, significantly impact blood sugar levels. The key lies in understanding how different foods affect you and planning meals accordingly.

Can a Vegetarian Diet Be Beneficial?

Recent research suggests a vegetarian diet, rich in whole grains, vegetables, legumes, and fruits, might offer some advantages for type 1 diabetics. Here's why:

- **Fiber Powerhouse:** Plant-based meals are typically high in fiber, which slows down carbohydrate digestion, leading to a steadier rise in blood sugar levels.
- **Weight Management:** Vegetarian diets often promote healthy weight management, another crucial factor in diabetes control.
- **Potential for Lower Insulin Needs:** Studies suggest a link between plant-based diets and reduced insulin requirements, although more research is needed.

Important Considerations:

- **Individualized Approach:** A vegetarian diet isn't a one-size-fits-all solution. Consult a registered dietitian to create a personalized plan that meets your specific needs and preferences. They can help you ensure you're getting enough essential nutrients like protein and healthy fats.

- **Carb Counting Remains Key:** Regardless of your dietary choices, understanding carbohydrate content in food is essential. This knowledge allows you to calculate insulin dosage effectively.

Beyond Food: Mastering Blood Sugar Levels

- **Blood Sugar Monitoring:** Regularly checking your blood sugar levels gives you valuable insights into how your body reacts to food, exercise, and stress.

- **Exercise – Your Reliable Partner:** Regular physical activity improves insulin sensitivity, helping your body utilize glucose more efficiently.

- **Stress Management:** Chronic stress can wreak havoc on blood sugar levels. Techniques like yoga or meditation can be powerful allies.

Remember: Living with Type 1 Diabetes requires a holistic approach, and adopting healthy lifestyle habits, you can take control and live a fulfilling life.

Chapter 1: 30 Day Meal Plan

Week 1:

Day 1:

- Breakfast: Avocado and Spinach Breakfast Bowl
- Lunch: Lentil Salad with Roasted Vegetables
- Dinner: Eggplant Parmesan
- Snack: Guacamole with Veggie Sticks
- Dessert: Berry Crisp with Oat Topping

Day 2:

- Breakfast: Vegetable Frittata
- Lunch: Chickpea Salad Sandwiches
- Dinner: Vegetarian Chili
- Snack: Hummus and Whole Wheat Pita Bread
- Dessert: Dark Chocolate Covered Strawberries

Day 3:

- Breakfast: Quinoa Breakfast Porridge
- Lunch: Caprese Salad with Balsamic Glaze
- Dinner: Spinach and Ricotta Stuffed Shells

- Snack: Cucumber and Tomato Bruschetta
- Dessert: Frozen Yogurt Bark with Mixed Berries

Day 4:

- Breakfast: Greek Yogurt Parfait with Berries
- Lunch: Vegetable Stir-Fry with Tofu
- Dinner: Mushroom and Spinach Quiche
- Snack: Edamame with Sea Salt
- Dessert: Banana Nice Cream

Day 5:

- Breakfast: Tofu Scramble with Vegetables
- Lunch: Quinoa Stuffed Bell Peppers
- Dinner: Cauliflower Curry with Brown Rice
- Snack: Roasted Chickpeas
- Dessert: Baked Apples with Cinnamon

Day 6:

- Breakfast: Oatmeal with Almond Butter and Banana
- Lunch: Greek Salad with Hummus Dressing
- Dinner: Ratatouille
- Snack: Greek Yogurt Dip with Fresh Vegetables

- Dessert: Lemon Poppy Seed Muffins

Day 7:

- Breakfast: Veggie Breakfast Burrito
- Lunch: Black Bean and Corn Quesadillas
- Dinner: Lentil Shepherd's Pie
- Snack: Stuffed Mini Bell Peppers
- Dessert: Chocolate Avocado Pudding

Week 2:

Day 8:

- Breakfast: Chia Seed Pudding with Almond Milk
- Lunch: Veggie Sushi Rolls
- Dinner: Veggie Stir-Fry with Brown Rice
- Snack: Avocado Slices on Whole Grain Crackers
- Dessert: Greek Yogurt Cheesecake with Berry Compote

Day 9:

- Breakfast: Sweet Potato and Black Bean Hash
- Lunch: Spinach and Strawberry Salad with Balsamic Vinaigrette

- Dinner: Eggplant and Zucchini Lasagna

- Snack: Baked Sweet Potato Fries

- Dessert: Coconut Macaroons

Day 10:

- Breakfast: Spinach and Mushroom Omelette

- Lunch: Mediterranean Veggie Wrap

- Dinner: Black Bean and Sweet Potato Tacos

- Snack: Caprese Skewers with Cherry Tomatoes and Mozzarella

- Dessert: Pumpkin Pie Smoothie Bowl

Day 11:

- Breakfast: Whole Wheat Pancakes with Sugar-Free Syrup

- Lunch: Cauliflower Fried Rice

- Dinner: Vegetable Paella

- Snack: Kale Chips

- Dessert: Chia Seed Jam on Whole Grain Toast

Day 12:

- Breakfast: Berry and Almond Smoothie Bowl

- Lunch: Tomato Basil Soup with Whole Grain Bread
- Dinner: Stuffed Acorn Squash with Quinoa and Cranberries
- Snack: Spinach and Artichoke Dip with Whole Grain Tortilla Chips
- Dessert: Oatmeal Raisin Cookies

Day 13:

- Breakfast: Zucchini and Carrot Muffins
- Lunch: Greek Chickpea Wraps
- Dinner: Thai Peanut Noodles with Tofu
- Snack: Greek Yogurt Bark with Berries and Nuts
- Dessert: Berry Parfait with Almond Granola

Day 14:

- Breakfast: Breakfast Quinoa with Fruit and Nuts
- Lunch: Butternut Squash and Kale Salad
- Dinner: Sweet Potato and Chickpea Curry
- Snack: Veggie Spring Rolls with Peanut Dipping Sauce
- Dessert: Mango Sorbet

Week 3:

Day 15:

- Breakfast: Vegan Breakfast Tacos
- Lunch: Broccoli and Cheese Stuffed Baked Potatoes
- Dinner: Mushroom Risotto
- Snack: Almond Butter and Apple Slices
- Dessert: Peanut Butter Energy Bites

Day 16:

- Breakfast: Avocado and Spinach Breakfast Bowl
- Lunch: Lentil Salad with Roasted Vegetables
- Dinner: Eggplant Parmesan
- Snack: Guacamole with Veggie Sticks
- Dessert: Berry Crisp with Oat Topping

Day 17:

- Breakfast: Vegetable Frittata
- Lunch: Chickpea Salad Sandwiches
- Dinner: Vegetarian Chili
- Snack: Hummus and Whole Wheat Pita Bread
- Dessert: Dark Chocolate Covered Strawberries

Day 18:

- Breakfast: Quinoa Breakfast Porridge
- Lunch: Caprese Salad with Balsamic Glaze
- Dinner: Spinach and Ricotta Stuffed Shells
- Snack: Cucumber and Tomato Bruschetta
- Dessert: Frozen Yogurt Bark with Mixed Berries

Day 19:

- Breakfast: Greek Yogurt Parfait with Berries
- Lunch: Vegetable Stir-Fry with Tofu
- Dinner: Mushroom and Spinach Quiche
- Snack: Edamame with Sea Salt
- Dessert: Banana Nice Cream

Day 20:

- Breakfast: Tofu Scramble with Vegetables
- Lunch: Quinoa Stuffed Bell Peppers
- Dinner: Cauliflower Curry with Brown Rice
- Snack: Roasted Chickpeas
- Dessert: Baked Apples with Cinnamon

Day 21:

- Breakfast: Oatmeal with Almond Butter and Banana
- Lunch: Greek Salad with Hummus Dressing
- Dinner: Ratatouille
- Snack: Greek Yogurt Dip with Fresh Vegetables
- Dessert: Lemon Poppy Seed Muffins

Day 22:

- Breakfast: Veggie Breakfast Burrito
- Lunch: Black Bean and Corn Quesadillas
- Dinner: Lentil Shepherd's Pie
- Snack: Stuffed Mini Bell Peppers
- Dessert: Chocolate Avocado Pudding

Day 23:

- Breakfast: Chia Seed Pudding with Almond Milk
- Lunch: Veggie Sushi Rolls
- Dinner: Veggie Stir-Fry with Brown Rice
- Snack: Avocado Slices on Whole Grain Crackers
- Dessert: Greek Yogurt Cheesecake with Berry Compote

Day 24:

- Breakfast: Sweet Potato and Black Bean Hash
- Lunch: Spinach and Strawberry Salad with Balsamic Vinaigrette
- Dinner: Eggplant and Zucchini Lasagna
- Snack: Baked Sweet Potato Fries
- Dessert: Coconut Macaroons

Day 25:

- Breakfast: Spinach and Mushroom Omelette
- Lunch: Mediterranean Veggie Wrap
- Dinner: Black Bean and Sweet Potato Tacos
- Snack: Caprese Skewers with Cherry Tomatoes and Mozzarella
- Dessert: Pumpkin Pie Smoothie Bowl

Day 26:

- Breakfast: Whole Wheat Pancakes with Sugar-Free Syrup
- Lunch: Cauliflower Fried Rice
- Dinner: Vegetable Paella
- Snack: Kale Chips

- Dessert: Chia Seed Jam on Whole Grain Toast

Day 27:

- Breakfast: Berry and Almond Smoothie Bowl
- Lunch: Tomato Basil Soup with Whole Grain Bread
- Dinner: Stuffed Acorn Squash with Quinoa and Cranberries
- Snack: Spinach and Artichoke Dip with Whole Grain Tortilla Chips
- Dessert: Oatmeal Raisin Cookies

Day 28:

- Breakfast: Zucchini and Carrot Muffins
- Lunch: Greek Chickpea Wraps
- Dinner: Thai Peanut Noodles with Tofu
- Snack: Greek Yogurt Bark with Berries and Nuts
- Dessert: Berry Parfait with Almond Granola

Day 29:

- Breakfast: Breakfast Quinoa with Fruit and Nuts
- Lunch: Butternut Squash and Kale Salad
- Dinner: Sweet Potato and Chickpea Curry

- Snack: Veggie Spring Rolls with Peanut Dipping Sauce
- Dessert: Mango Sorbet

Day 30:

- Breakfast: Vegan Breakfast Tacos
- Lunch: Broccoli and Cheese Stuffed Baked Potatoes
- Dinner: Mushroom Risotto
- Snack: Almond Butter and Apple Slices
- Dessert: Peanut Butter Energy Bites

Chapter 2: Breakfast Recipes

Breakfast is often hailed as the most important meal of the day, especially for those managing their health, including individuals with Type 1 diabetes. In this chapter, we present a variety of nutritious and delicious breakfast recipes tailored for Type 1 diabetics.

Avocado and Spinach Breakfast Bowl

Ingredients:

- 1 ripe avocado
- 1 cup fresh spinach leaves
- 1/4 cup cherry tomatoes, halved
- 1/4 cup diced red bell pepper
- 1 tablespoon lemon juice
- Salt and pepper to taste

Instructions:

1. Mash the avocado in a bowl until smooth.

2. Stir in the spinach, cherry tomatoes, red bell pepper, and lemon juice.
3. Season with salt and pepper.
4. Serve in a bowl and enjoy!

Nutrition Information:

- Calories: 250
- Protein: 5g
- Carbohydrates: 15g
- Fat: 20g
- Fiber: 9g
- Sugar: 2g
- Portion Size: 1 bowl

Vegetable Frittata

Ingredients:

- 6 large eggs
- 1/4 cup diced onion
- 1/4 cup diced bell peppers
- 1/4 cup diced zucchini
- 1/4 cup diced mushrooms
- Salt and pepper to taste

Instructions:

1. Preheat your oven to 350°F (175°C).
2. In a bowl, whisk together the eggs, salt, and pepper.
3. Heat an oven-safe skillet over medium heat and add a little oil.
4. Sauté the onions, bell peppers, zucchini, and mushrooms until softened.
5. Pour the whisked eggs over the vegetables in the skillet.
6. Cook for 2-3 minutes until the edges start to set.
7. Transfer the skillet to the oven and bake for 10-12 minutes until the frittata is cooked through.
8. Slice and serve!

Nutrition Information:

- Calories: 180
- Protein: 14g
- Carbohydrates: 5g
- Fat: 11g
- Fiber: 1g
- Sugar: 2g
- Portion Size: 1 slice

Quinoa Breakfast Porridge

Ingredients:

- 1/2 cup quinoa, rinsed
- 1 cup almond milk
- 1/2 teaspoon cinnamon
- 1 tablespoon maple syrup
- 1/4 cup chopped nuts (such as almonds or walnuts)
- Fresh berries for topping

Instructions:

1. In a saucepan, combine the quinoa and almond milk.
2. Bring to a boil, then reduce heat and simmer for 15-20 minutes until quinoa is cooked and liquid is absorbed.
3. Stir in the cinnamon and maple syrup.
4. Serve hot, topped with chopped nuts and fresh berries.

Nutrition Information:

- Calories: 280
- Protein: 9g
- Carbohydrates: 40g

- Fat: 10g
- Fiber: 6g
- Sugar: 8g
- Portion Size: 1 serving

Greek Yogurt Parfait with Berries

Ingredients:
- 1/2 cup Greek yogurt
- 1/4 cup granola
- 1/4 cup mixed berries (such as strawberries, blueberries, and raspberries)
- Drizzle of honey (optional)

Instructions:
1. In a glass or bowl, layer Greek yogurt, granola, and mixed berries.
2. Repeat layers until ingredients are used up.
3. Drizzle with honey if desired.
4. Serve immediately and enjoy!

Nutrition Information:
- Calories: 200

- Protein: 10g

- Carbohydrates: 30g

- Fat: 5g

- Fiber: 5g

- Sugar: 12g

- Portion Size: 1 serving

Tofu Scramble with Vegetables

Ingredients:

- 1/2 block firm tofu, crumbled

- 1/4 cup diced onion

- 1/4 cup diced bell peppers

- 1/4 cup diced tomatoes

- 1/2 teaspoon turmeric

- Salt and pepper to taste

Instructions:

1. Heat a skillet over medium heat and add a little oil.

2. Sauté the onions, bell peppers, and tomatoes until softened.

3. Add the crumbled tofu to the skillet.

4. Season with turmeric, salt, and pepper.

5. Cook for 5-7 minutes until tofu is heated through.

6. Serve hot and enjoy!

Nutrition Information:

- Calories: 180

- Protein: 15g

- Carbohydrates: 10g

- Fat: 10g

- Fiber: 3g

- Sugar: 4g

- Portion Size: 1 serving

Oatmeal with Almond Butter and Banana

Ingredients:

- 1/2 cup rolled oats

- 1 cup water or milk of choice

- 1 tablespoon almond butter

- 1/2 banana, sliced

- Drizzle of honey (optional)

Instructions:

1. In a saucepan, bring the water or milk to a boil.
2. Stir in the rolled oats and reduce heat to low.
3. Cook for 5-7 minutes, stirring occasionally, until oats are creamy.
4. Transfer oatmeal to a bowl and top with almond butter and banana slices.
5. Drizzle with honey if desired.
6. Serve hot and enjoy!

Nutrition Information:

- Calories: 300
- Protein: 8g
- Carbohydrates: 45g
- Fat: 10g
- Fiber: 7g
- Sugar: 12g
- Portion Size: 1 serving

Veggie Breakfast Burrito

Ingredients:

- 1 whole wheat tortilla

- 2 scrambled eggs
- 1/4 cup black beans
- 1/4 cup diced bell peppers
- 1/4 cup diced tomatoes
- Salsa or hot sauce for topping

Instructions:

1. Warm the tortilla in a skillet or microwave.
2. Layer the scrambled eggs, black beans, bell peppers, and tomatoes in the center of the tortilla.
3. Fold in the sides of the tortilla, then roll it up tightly.
4. Heat the burrito in the skillet for 1-2 minutes on each side until lightly browned.
5. Serve with salsa or hot sauce on top.
6. Enjoy your delicious breakfast burrito!

Nutrition Information:

- Calories: 320
- Protein: 20g
- Carbohydrates: 35g
- Fat: 12g
- Fiber: 8g

- Sugar: 3g
- Portion Size: 1 burrito

Chia Seed Pudding with Almond Milk

Ingredients:

- 1/4 cup chia seeds
- 1 cup almond milk
- 1/2 teaspoon vanilla extract
- Fresh fruit for topping (such as berries or sliced mango)

Instructions:

1. In a bowl, combine the chia seeds, almond milk, and vanilla extract.
2. Stir well to combine, then cover and refrigerate for at least 2 hours or overnight.
3. Once the pudding has set, give it a good stir.
4. Serve in a bowl or jar, topped with fresh fruit.
5. Enjoy your nutritious chia seed pudding!

Nutrition Information:

- Calories: 180

- Protein: 6g

- Carbohydrates: 20g

- Fat: 9g

- Fiber: 10g

- Sugar: 4g

- Portion Size: 1 serving

Sweet Potato and Black Bean Hash

Ingredients:

- 1 medium sweet potato, diced

- 1/2 cup black beans, drained and rinsed

- 1/4 cup diced onion

- 1/4 cup diced bell peppers

- 1 teaspoon cumin

- Salt and pepper to taste

Instructions:

1. Heat a skillet over medium heat and add a little oil.

2. Add the diced sweet potato to the skillet and cook for 5-7 minutes until slightly tender.

3. Add the black beans, onion, and bell peppers to the skillet.

4. Season with cumin, salt, and pepper.

5. Cook for another 5 minutes until vegetables are cooked through and flavors are combined.

6. Serve hot and enjoy!

Nutrition Information:

- Calories: 220
- Protein: 8g
- Carbohydrates: 40g
- Fat: 3g
- Fiber: 9g
- Sugar: 6g
- Portion Size: 1 serving

Spinach and Mushroom Omelette

Ingredients:

- 2 eggs
- 1/4 cup fresh spinach leaves
- 1/4 cup sliced mushrooms
- 2 tablespoons shredded cheese (optional)
- Salt and pepper to taste

Instructions:

1. Crack the eggs into a bowl and whisk until well beaten.
2. Heat a non-stick skillet over medium heat and add a little oil.
3. Pour the beaten eggs into the skillet.
4. Scatter the spinach leaves and sliced mushrooms over one half of the omelette.
5. If using cheese, sprinkle it over the vegetables.
6. Season with salt and pepper.
7. Cook for 2-3 minutes until the edges start to set.
8. Carefully fold the omelette in half with a spatula.
9. Cook for another 1-2 minutes until cooked through.
10. Slide onto a plate and serve hot.

Nutrition Information:

- Calories: 250
- Protein: 18g
- Carbohydrates: 5g
- Fat: 18g
- Fiber: 2g
- Sugar: 2g

- Portion Size: 1 serving

Whole Wheat Pancakes with Sugar-Free Syrup

Ingredients:

- 1/2 cup whole wheat flour
- 1/2 teaspoon baking powder
- 1/4 teaspoon cinnamon
- 1/2 cup almond milk
- 1 tablespoon maple syrup (or sugar-free syrup)
- 1/2 teaspoon vanilla extract

Instructions:

1. In a bowl, whisk together the whole wheat flour, baking powder, and cinnamon.
2. Stir in the almond milk, maple syrup, and vanilla extract until well combined.
3. Heat a non-stick skillet over medium heat and lightly grease with oil.
4. Pour about 1/4 cup of batter onto the skillet for each pancake.

5. Cook for 2-3 minutes until bubbles form on the surface, then flip and cook for another 1-2 minutes until golden brown.

6. Serve hot with sugar-free syrup.

Nutrition Information:

- Calories: 200
- Protein: 5g
- Carbohydrates: 35g
- Fat: 4g
- Fiber: 5g
- Sugar: 3g
- Portion Size: 2 pancakes

Berry and Almond Smoothie Bowl

Ingredients:

- 1/2 cup mixed berries (such as strawberries, blueberries, and raspberries)
- 1/2 banana
- 1/4 cup almond milk
- 1 tablespoon almond butter
- 1 tablespoon chia seeds

- Toppings: sliced almonds, shredded coconut, additional berries

Instructions:

1. In a blender, combine the mixed berries, banana, almond milk, almond butter, and chia seeds.
2. Blend until smooth and creamy.
3. Pour the smoothie into a bowl.
4. Top with sliced almonds, shredded coconut, and additional berries.
5. Serve immediately and enjoy!

Nutrition Information:

- Calories: 300
- Protein: 7g
- Carbohydrates: 35g
- Fat: 15g
- Fiber: 10g
- Sugar: 15g
- Portion Size: 1 serving

Zucchini and Carrot Muffins

Ingredients:

- 1 cup grated zucchini
- 1/2 cup grated carrot
- 1/4 cup unsweetened applesauce
- 1/4 cup maple syrup
- 1/4 cup almond milk
- 1 teaspoon vanilla extract
- 1 cup whole wheat flour
- 1/2 teaspoon baking powder
- 1/2 teaspoon baking soda
- 1/2 teaspoon cinnamon
- Pinch of salt
- 1/4 cup chopped nuts (optional)

Instructions:

1. Preheat your oven to 350°F (175°C) and line a muffin tin with liners or grease with oil.
2. In a bowl, combine the grated zucchini, grated carrot, applesauce, maple syrup, almond milk, and vanilla extract.

3. In another bowl, whisk together the whole wheat flour, baking powder, baking soda, cinnamon, and salt.

4. Pour the wet ingredients into the dry ingredients and stir until just combined.

5. Fold in the chopped nuts if using.

6. Divide the batter evenly among the muffin cups.

7. Bake for 20-25 minutes until golden brown and a toothpick inserted into the center comes out clean.

8. Allow muffins to cool in the tin for 5 minutes before transferring to a wire rack to cool completely.

9. Enjoy these delicious muffins for breakfast or as a snack!

Nutrition Information:
- Calories: 150
- Protein: 4g
- Carbohydrates: 25g
- Fat: 5g
- Fiber: 3g
- Sugar: 10g
- Portion Size: 1 muffin

Breakfast Quinoa with Fruit and Nuts

Ingredients:

- 1/2 cup cooked quinoa
- 1/4 cup almond milk
- 1/4 teaspoon cinnamon
- 1/4 cup mixed fresh fruit (such as berries, sliced banana, and diced apple)
- 1 tablespoon chopped nuts (such as almonds or walnuts)
- Drizzle of honey or maple syrup (optional)

Instructions:

1. In a saucepan, warm the cooked quinoa with almond milk and cinnamon over low heat.
2. Stir until heated through and creamy.
3. Transfer the quinoa to a bowl and top with mixed fresh fruit and chopped nuts.
4. Drizzle with honey or maple syrup if desired.
5. Serve warm and enjoy this nutritious breakfast!

Nutrition Information:

- Calories: 220
- Protein: 6g
- Carbohydrates: 35g
- Fat: 6g
- Fiber: 5g
- Sugar: 10g
- Portion Size: 1 serving

Vegan Breakfast Tacos

Ingredients:

- 4 small corn tortillas
- 1/2 cup black beans, drained and rinsed
- 1/2 avocado, sliced
- 1/4 cup salsa
- Fresh cilantro for garnish
- Lime wedges for serving

Instructions:

1. Warm the corn tortillas in a dry skillet over medium heat for about 30 seconds on each side until soft and pliable.

2. Heat the black beans in a small saucepan over low heat until heated through.

3. To assemble the tacos, divide the black beans evenly among the tortillas.

4. Top each taco with sliced avocado, salsa, and fresh cilantro.

5. Serve with lime wedges on the side for squeezing over the tacos.

6. Enjoy these flavorful vegan breakfast tacos to start your day off right!

Nutrition Information:

- Calories: 200
- Protein: 6g
- Carbohydrates: 30g
- Fat: 8g
- Fiber: 8g
- Sugar: 2g
- Portion Size: 2 tacos

Chapter 3: Lunch Recipes

Lunchtime offers an opportunity to refuel and recharge your body midday. These lunch recipes are not only delicious but also packed with nutrients to keep you energized throughout the day. From salads to wraps to hearty soups, there's something here to satisfy every craving.

Lentil Salad with Roasted Vegetables

Ingredients:

- 1 cup cooked lentils
- Assorted vegetables (e.g., bell peppers, zucchini, cherry tomatoes)
- Olive oil
- Balsamic vinegar
- Salt and pepper to taste

Instructions:

1. Preheat oven to 400°F (200°C).

2. Toss vegetables with olive oil, salt, and pepper, then spread on a baking sheet.

3. Roast vegetables for 20-25 minutes until tender.

4. In a bowl, combine cooked lentils and roasted vegetables.

5. Drizzle with balsamic vinegar and toss to coat.

6. Serve warm or chilled.

Nutrition Information:

- Calories: 250
- Protein: 12g
- Carbohydrates: 40g
- Fat: 5g
- Fiber: 10g
- Sugar: 5g
- Portion Size: 1 serving

Chickpea Salad Sandwiches

Ingredients:

- 1 can chickpeas, drained and rinsed
- Celery, diced
- Red onion, diced

- Vegan mayonnaise
- Dijon mustard
- Whole grain bread
- Lettuce leaves

Instructions:

1. In a bowl, mash chickpeas with a fork.
2. Add diced celery, red onion, vegan mayonnaise, and Dijon mustard. Mix well.
3. Spread chickpea salad on whole grain bread.
4. Top with lettuce leaves and another slice of bread.
5. Serve as sandwiches.

Nutrition Information:

- Calories: 300
- Protein: 15g
- Carbohydrates: 45g
- Fat: 8g
- Fiber: 10g
- Sugar: 5g
- Portion Size: 1 sandwich

Caprese Salad with Balsamic Glaze

Ingredients:

- Fresh mozzarella cheese, sliced
- Tomatoes, sliced
- Fresh basil leaves
- Balsamic glaze
- Salt and pepper to taste

Instructions:

1. Arrange alternating slices of mozzarella cheese and tomatoes on a plate.
2. Tuck fresh basil leaves between cheese and tomatoes.
3. Drizzle with balsamic glaze.
4. Season with salt and pepper to taste.

Nutrition Information:

- Calories: 200
- Protein: 12g
- Carbohydrates: 8g
- Fat: 15g
- Fiber: 2g

- Sugar: 5g
- Portion Size: 1 serving

Vegetable Stir-Fry with Tofu

Ingredients:

- Firm tofu, cubed
- Assorted vegetables (e.g., bell peppers, broccoli, carrots, snap peas)
- Soy sauce
- Garlic, minced
- Ginger, grated
- Sesame oil
- Cooked brown rice or quinoa (optional)

Instructions:

1. Heat sesame oil in a large skillet or wok over medium-high heat.
2. Add tofu cubes and cook until golden brown on all sides. Remove from skillet and set aside.
3. In the same skillet, add minced garlic and grated ginger. Cook until fragrant.

4. Add assorted vegetables to the skillet and stir-fry until tender-crisp.

5. Return tofu to the skillet and add soy sauce.

6. Cook for another 2-3 minutes, stirring occasionally.

7. Serve hot over cooked brown rice or quinoa if desired.

Nutrition Information:

- Calories: 300
- Protein: 20g
- Carbohydrates: 25g
- Fat: 15g
- Fiber: 8g
- Sugar: 5g
- Portion Size: 1 serving

Quinoa Stuffed Bell Peppers

Ingredients:

- Bell peppers, halved and seeds removed
- Cooked quinoa
- Black beans, drained and rinsed
- Corn kernels

- Diced tomatoes
- Mexican seasoning blend
- Shredded cheese (optional)

Instructions:

1. Preheat oven to 375°F (190°C).
2. In a bowl, mix cooked quinoa, black beans, corn kernels, diced tomatoes, and Mexican seasoning blend.
3. Stuff each bell pepper half with the quinoa mixture.
4. Place stuffed bell peppers in a baking dish.
5. If desired, sprinkle shredded cheese on top.
6. Bake for 25-30 minutes until bell peppers are tender.
7. Serve hot.

Nutrition Information:

- Calories: 280
- Protein: 15g
- Carbohydrates: 40g
- Fat: 8g
- Fiber: 10g
- Sugar: 5g

- Portion Size: 1 stuffed bell pepper half

Greek Salad with Hummus Dressing

Ingredients:

- Cucumber, diced
- Cherry tomatoes, halved
- Kalamata olives, pitted
- Red onion, thinly sliced
- Feta cheese, crumbled
- Hummus
- Lemon juice
- Dried oregano
- Olive oil
- Salt and pepper to taste

Instructions:

1. In a large bowl, combine diced cucumber, halved cherry tomatoes, Kalamata olives, sliced red onion, and crumbled feta cheese.

2. In a small bowl, whisk together hummus, lemon juice, dried oregano, olive oil, salt, and pepper to make the dressing.

3. Drizzle the hummus dressing over the salad and toss to coat.

4. Serve chilled.

Nutrition Information:

- Calories: 220
- Protein: 10g
- Carbohydrates: 15g
- Fat: 15g
- Fiber: 5g
- Sugar: 5g
- Portion Size: 1 serving

Black Bean and Corn Quesadillas

Ingredients:

- Whole grain tortillas
- Black beans, drained and rinsed
- Corn kernels
- Shredded cheese (use reduced-fat if desired)
- Salsa
- Avocado slices (optional)

Instructions:

1. Heat a non-stick skillet over medium heat.

2. Place a tortilla in the skillet and spread black beans and corn kernels evenly over half of the tortilla.

3. Sprinkle shredded cheese over the beans and corn.

4. Fold the other half of the tortilla over the filling to form a half-moon shape.

5. Cook until the bottom is golden brown, then flip and cook the other side until golden brown and the cheese is melted.

6. Repeat with remaining tortillas and filling.

7. Serve hot with salsa and avocado slices if desired.

Nutrition Information:

- Calories: 280
- Protein: 15g
- Carbohydrates: 35g
- Fat: 10g
- Fiber: 8g
- Sugar: 5g
- Portion Size: 1 quesadilla

Veggie Sushi Rolls

Ingredients:

- Sushi rice
- Nori seaweed sheets
- Assorted vegetables (e.g., cucumber, avocado, carrot, bell pepper)
- Soy sauce
- Pickled ginger
- Wasabi (optional)

Instructions:

1. Cook sushi rice according to package instructions and let cool.
2. Place a nori seaweed sheet on a bamboo sushi mat.
3. Spread a thin layer of sushi rice over the nori, leaving a 1-inch border at the top.
4. Arrange thinly sliced vegetables in the center of the rice.
5. Using the bamboo mat, roll the nori tightly into a cylinder.
6. Slice the roll into bite-sized pieces using a sharp knife.

7. Serve with soy sauce, pickled ginger, and wasabi if desired.

Nutrition Information:

- Calories: 250
- Protein: 8g
- Carbohydrates: 50g
- Fat: 2g
- Fiber: 5g
- Sugar: 5g
- Portion Size: 1 serving (4-6 sushi rolls)

Spinach and Strawberry Salad with Balsamic Vinaigrette

Ingredients:

- Fresh spinach leaves
- Fresh strawberries, sliced
- Red onion, thinly sliced
- Feta cheese, crumbled
- Balsamic vinaigrette dressing

Instructions:

1. In a large bowl, combine fresh spinach leaves, sliced strawberries, sliced red onion, and crumbled feta cheese.
2. Drizzle with balsamic vinaigrette dressing and toss to coat evenly.
3. Serve immediately.

Nutrition Information:

- Calories: 180
- Protein: 5g
- Carbohydrates: 20g
- Fat: 10g
- Fiber: 5g
- Sugar: 10g
- Portion Size: 1 serving

Mediterranean Veggie Wrap

Ingredients:

- Whole grain wrap
- Hummus
- Baby spinach leaves

- Sliced cucumber

- Sliced tomatoes

- Sliced red bell pepper

- Sliced red onion

- Kalamata olives, pitted

- Feta cheese, crumbled (optional)

Instructions:

1. Spread a layer of hummus on a whole grain wrap.

2. Layer baby spinach leaves, sliced cucumber, sliced tomatoes, sliced red bell pepper, sliced red onion, and Kalamata olives on top of the hummus.

3. If desired, sprinkle crumbled feta cheese over the vegetables.

4. Roll up the wrap tightly, tucking in the sides as you go.

5. Slice the wrap in half and serve.

Nutrition Information:

- Calories: 300

- Protein: 10g

- Carbohydrates: 40g

- Fat: 12g

- Fiber: 8g

- Sugar: 5g

- Portion Size: 1 wrap

Cauliflower Fried Rice

Ingredients:

- Cauliflower rice

- Mixed vegetables (e.g., carrots, peas, corn)

- Eggs

- Soy sauce

- Garlic powder

- Sesame oil

- Green onions, chopped

Instructions:

1. Heat sesame oil in a large skillet or wok over medium heat.

2. Add mixed vegetables and cook until tender.

3. Push vegetables to one side of the skillet and crack eggs into the empty space.

4. Scramble eggs until cooked through, then mix with the vegetables.

5. Add cauliflower rice to the skillet and stir-fry until heated through.

6. Season with soy sauce, garlic powder, and chopped green onions.

7. Cook for another 2-3 minutes, stirring constantly.

8. Serve hot.

Nutrition Information:

- Calories: 200
- Protein: 10g
- Carbohydrates: 25g
- Fat: 8g
- Fiber: 8g
- Sugar: 5g
- Portion Size: 1 serving

Tomato Basil Soup with Whole Grain Bread

Ingredients:

- Canned diced tomatoes
- Vegetable broth
- Fresh basil leaves
- Garlic, minced
- Onion, diced
- Olive oil
- Whole grain bread slices

Instructions:

1. Heat olive oil in a large pot over medium heat.
2. Add minced garlic and diced onion. Cook until softened.
3. Pour in canned diced tomatoes and vegetable broth.
4. Bring to a simmer and let cook for 15-20 minutes.
5. Stir in fresh basil leaves and season with salt and pepper to taste.
6. Use an immersion blender to blend the soup until smooth.
7. Serve hot with whole grain bread slices.

Nutrition Information:

- Calories: 180
- Protein: 5g
- Carbohydrates: 30g
- Fat: 5g
- Fiber: 8g
- Sugar: 10g
- Portion Size: 1 serving

Greek Chickpea Wraps

Ingredients:

- Whole grain wrap
- Chickpeas, cooked or canned
- Cherry tomatoes, halved
- Cucumber, diced
- Red onion, thinly sliced
- Kalamata olives, pitted and sliced
- Feta cheese, crumbled
- Greek yogurt
- Lemon juice
- Dried oregano
- Salt and pepper to taste

Instructions:

1. In a bowl, mix together chickpeas, cherry tomatoes, cucumber, red onion, Kalamata olives, and crumbled feta cheese.
2. In a separate small bowl, mix Greek yogurt with lemon juice, dried oregano, salt, and pepper to make the dressing.
3. Spread a layer of the Greek yogurt dressing onto a whole grain wrap.
4. Spoon the chickpea mixture onto the wrap.
5. Roll up the wrap tightly and slice in half.
6. Serve immediately.

Nutrition Information:

- Calories: 280
- Protein: 10g
- Carbohydrates: 35g
- Fat: 10g
- Fiber: 8g
- Sugar: 5g
- Portion Size: 1 wrap

Butternut Squash and Kale Salad

Ingredients:

- Butternut squash, diced
- Kale leaves, stems removed and chopped
- Dried cranberries
- Toasted pecans, chopped
- Goat cheese, crumbled
- Balsamic vinaigrette dressing

Instructions:

1. Preheat oven to 400°F (200°C).
2. Toss diced butternut squash with olive oil, salt, and pepper.
3. Spread on a baking sheet and roast for 20-25 minutes until tender.
4. In a large bowl, combine roasted butternut squash, chopped kale leaves, dried cranberries, toasted pecans, and crumbled goat cheese.
5. Drizzle with balsamic vinaigrette dressing and toss to coat.
6. Serve chilled or at room temperature.

Nutrition Information:

- Calories: 250
- Protein: 8g
- Carbohydrates: 30g
- Fat: 12g
- Fiber: 8g
- Sugar: 10g
- Portion Size: 1 serving

Broccoli and Cheese Stuffed Baked Potatoes

Ingredients:

- Russet potatoes
- Broccoli florets, steamed
- Shredded cheddar cheese
- Greek yogurt or sour cream
- Chives, chopped
- Salt and pepper to taste

Instructions:

1. Preheat oven to 400°F (200°C).

2. Scrub potatoes and pierce with a fork.

3. Bake potatoes for 45-60 minutes until tender.

4. Cut a slit in the top of each potato and fluff the insides with a fork.

5. Stuff each potato with steamed broccoli florets and shredded cheddar cheese.

6. Return to the oven for 5-10 minutes until cheese is melted.

7. Top with Greek yogurt or sour cream, chopped chives, salt, and pepper.

8. Serve hot.

Nutrition Information:

- Calories: 300
- Protein: 10g
- Carbohydrates: 40g
- Fat: 10g
- Fiber: 8g
- Sugar: 5g
- Portion Size: 1 baked potato

Chapter 4: Dinner Recipes

These dinner recipes are not only packed with flavor but are also carefully crafted to provide balanced nutrition suitable for individuals managing Type 1 diabetes. From comforting classics to exotic flavors, there's something for everyone to enjoy while keeping blood sugar levels in check.

Eggplant Parmesan

Ingredients:

- 1 large eggplant
- 1 cup breadcrumbs
- 1 cup marinara sauce
- 1 cup shredded mozzarella cheese
- 1/4 cup grated Parmesan cheese
- Fresh basil leaves for garnish

Instructions:

1. Preheat oven to 375°F (190°C).
2. Slice eggplant into 1/4-inch rounds.

3. Dip eggplant slices in breadcrumbs, coating both sides.

4. Place coated eggplant slices on a baking sheet and bake for 15-20 minutes until golden brown.

5. In a baking dish, spread a layer of marinara sauce, then layer baked eggplant slices.

6. Top with remaining marinara sauce, mozzarella, and Parmesan cheese.

7. Bake for an additional 20-25 minutes until cheese is melted and bubbly.

8. Garnish with fresh basil leaves before serving.

Nutrition Information (per serving):

- Calories: 280
- Protein: 12g
- Carbohydrates: 30g
- Fat: 12g
- Fiber: 6g
- Sugar: 8g
- Portion size: 1/6 of recipe

Vegetarian Chili

Ingredients:

- 1 can (15 oz) black beans, drained and rinsed
- 1 can (15 oz) kidney beans, drained and rinsed
- 1 can (15 oz) diced tomatoes
- 1 onion, diced
- 2 cloves garlic, minced
- 1 bell pepper, diced
- 1 cup corn kernels
- 2 tablespoons chili powder
- 1 teaspoon cumin
- Salt and pepper to taste
- Optional toppings: shredded cheese, chopped cilantro, diced avocado

Instructions:

1. In a large pot, sauté onion, garlic, and bell pepper until softened.
2. Add beans, diced tomatoes, corn, chili powder, cumin, salt, and pepper.
3. Bring to a simmer and let cook for 20-25 minutes.
4. Serve hot, topped with optional toppings if desired.

Nutrition Information (per serving):

- Calories: 250
- Protein: 12g
- Carbohydrates: 45g
- Fat: 2g
- Fiber: 14g
- Sugar: 8g
- Portion size: 1/6 of recipe

Spinach and Ricotta Stuffed Shells

Ingredients:

- 1 box (12 oz) jumbo pasta shells
- 2 cups ricotta cheese
- 1 cup chopped spinach
- 1/2 cup grated Parmesan cheese
- 1 egg
- 1 teaspoon dried oregano
- Salt and pepper to taste
- 2 cups marinara sauce
- 1 cup shredded mozzarella cheese

Instructions:

1. Cook pasta shells according to package instructions until al dente. Drain and set aside.

2. In a bowl, mix together ricotta cheese, chopped spinach, Parmesan cheese, egg, oregano, salt, and pepper.

3. Preheat oven to 375°F (190°C).

4. Stuff cooked pasta shells with ricotta mixture and place in a baking dish.

5. Pour marinara sauce over stuffed shells and sprinkle with mozzarella cheese.

6. Cover with foil and bake for 25-30 minutes, then uncover and bake for an additional 10 minutes until cheese is melted and bubbly.

7. Serve hot.

Nutrition Information (per serving):

- Calories: 320

- Protein: 18g

- Carbohydrates: 35g

- Fat: 12g

- Fiber: 4g

- Sugar: 6g
- Portion size: 2 stuffed shells

Mushroom and Spinach Quiche

Ingredients:

- 1 pie crust (store-bought or homemade)
- 1 cup sliced mushrooms
- 2 cups fresh spinach
- 1 onion, diced
- 4 eggs
- 1 cup milk (or non-dairy alternative)
- 1/2 cup shredded cheese (optional)
- Salt and pepper to taste

Instructions:

1. Preheat oven to 375°F (190°C).
2. In a skillet, sauté mushrooms, spinach, and onion until softened.
3. In a bowl, whisk together eggs, milk, salt, and pepper.
4. Place pie crust in a pie dish and spread mushroom-spinach mixture evenly on the bottom.

5. Pour egg mixture over the vegetables.

6. Sprinkle shredded cheese on top if desired.

7. Bake for 35-40 minutes until the center is set and the crust is golden brown.

8. Let cool slightly before slicing and serving.

Nutrition Information (per serving):

- Calories: 280

- Protein: 14g

- Carbohydrates: 20g

- Fat: 16g

- Fiber: 2g

- Sugar: 4g

- Portion size: 1/6 of quiche

Cauliflower Curry with Brown Rice

Ingredients:

- 1 head cauliflower, chopped into florets

- 1 onion, diced

- 2 cloves garlic, minced

- 1 tablespoon curry powder

- 1 can (15 oz) chickpeas, drained and rinsed

- 1 can (14 oz) coconut milk
- 1 cup vegetable broth
- 2 cups cooked brown rice
- Fresh cilantro for garnish
- Salt and pepper to taste

Instructions:

1. In a large skillet, sauté onion and garlic until fragrant.
2. Add cauliflower florets and curry powder, stirring to coat.
3. Pour in coconut milk and vegetable broth, then add chickpeas.
4. Bring to a simmer and cook for 15-20 minutes until cauliflower is tender.
5. Season with salt and pepper to taste.
6. Serve over cooked brown rice, garnished with fresh cilantro.

Nutrition Information (per serving):

- Calories: 350
- Protein: 10g
- Carbohydrates: 45g

- Fat: 15g

- Fiber: 8g

- Sugar: 6g

- Portion size: 1/4 of recipe

Ratatouille

Ingredients:

- 1 eggplant, diced

- 2 zucchinis, diced

- 1 bell pepper, diced

- 1 onion, diced

- 2 cloves garlic, minced

- 2 cups diced tomatoes

- 1 tablespoon olive oil

- 1 teaspoon dried thyme

- Salt and pepper to taste

- Fresh basil for garnish

Instructions:

1. Preheat oven to 375°F (190°C).

2. In a large baking dish, toss together diced eggplant, zucchini, bell pepper, onion, and garlic.

3. Drizzle with olive oil and sprinkle with dried thyme, salt, and pepper. Toss to coat.

4. Bake for 25-30 minutes until vegetables are tender.

5. Serve hot, garnished with fresh basil.

Nutrition Information (per serving):

- Calories: 180
- Protein: 4g
- Carbohydrates: 25g
- Fat: 8g
- Fiber: 8g
- Sugar: 12g
- Portion size: 1/4 of recipe

Lentil Shepherd's Pie

Ingredients:

- 1 cup dry green lentils
- 2 cups vegetable broth
- 1 onion, diced
- 2 carrots, diced
- 2 cloves garlic, minced
- 1 cup frozen peas

- 2 tablespoons tomato paste
- 1 teaspoon dried thyme
- Mashed potatoes (prepared separately)
- Salt and pepper to taste

Instructions:

1. Preheat oven to 375°F (190°C).
2. In a pot, combine lentils and vegetable broth. Bring to a boil, then reduce heat and simmer for 20-25 minutes until lentils are tender and most of the liquid is absorbed.
3. In a skillet, sauté onion, carrots, and garlic until softened.
4. Add cooked lentils, frozen peas, tomato paste, and dried thyme to the skillet. Stir to combine.
5. Season with salt and pepper to taste.
6. Transfer lentil mixture to a baking dish.
7. Spread mashed potatoes over the top to cover the lentil mixture completely.
8. Bake for 25-30 minutes until the mashed potatoes are golden brown.
9. Serve hot.

Nutrition Information (per serving):

- Calories: 320
- Protein: 14g
- Carbohydrates: 60g
- Fat: 2g
- Fiber: 16g
- Sugar: 8g
- Portion size: 1/6 of recipe

Veggie Stir-Fry with Brown Rice

Ingredients:

- 2 cups cooked brown rice
- 1 bell pepper, thinly sliced
- 1 cup broccoli florets
- 1 carrot, thinly sliced
- 1 cup snap peas
- 1/2 cup sliced mushrooms
- 2 cloves garlic, minced
- 2 tablespoons soy sauce
- 1 tablespoon sesame oil
- Optional toppings: chopped green onions, sesame seeds

Instructions:

1. Heat sesame oil in a large skillet over medium heat.

2. Add garlic and sauté until fragrant.

3. Add bell pepper, broccoli, carrot, snap peas, and mushrooms to the skillet. Stir-fry for 5-7 minutes until vegetables are tender-crisp.

4. Stir in cooked brown rice and soy sauce, tossing to combine.

5. Cook for an additional 2-3 minutes until heated through.

6. Serve hot, topped with optional green onions and sesame seeds.

Nutrition Information (per serving):

- Calories: 280
- Protein: 8g
- Carbohydrates: 50g
- Fat: 6g
- Fiber: 10g
- Sugar: 6g
- Portion size: 1/4 of recipe

Eggplant and Zucchini Lasagna

Ingredients:

- 1 large eggplant, sliced lengthwise
- 2 medium zucchinis, sliced lengthwise
- 2 cups marinara sauce
- 2 cups ricotta cheese
- 1 cup shredded mozzarella cheese
- 1/4 cup grated Parmesan cheese
- 1 teaspoon dried basil
- Salt and pepper to taste

Instructions:

1. Preheat oven to 375°F (190°C).
2. Lightly salt eggplant and zucchini slices and let sit for 10 minutes to release excess moisture. Pat dry with paper towels.
3. In a baking dish, spread a thin layer of marinara sauce.
4. Layer eggplant slices, followed by ricotta cheese, zucchini slices, and more marinara sauce. Repeat until all ingredients are used, ending with a layer of marinara sauce on top.

5. Sprinkle mozzarella and Parmesan cheese over the top.

6. Cover with foil and bake for 30 minutes.

7. Remove foil and bake for an additional 15-20 minutes until cheese is bubbly and golden.

8. Let cool slightly before serving.

Nutrition Information (per serving):

- Calories: 280
- Protein: 15g
- Carbohydrates: 20g
- Fat: 15g
- Fiber: 6g
- Sugar: 8g
- Portion size: 1/6 of recipe

Black Bean and Sweet Potato Tacos

Ingredients:

- 1 can (15 oz) black beans, drained and rinsed
- 2 medium sweet potatoes, peeled and diced
- 1 onion, diced
- 2 cloves garlic, minced

- 1 tablespoon chili powder
- 1 teaspoon cumin
- 1 teaspoon paprika
- Salt and pepper to taste
- 8 small whole wheat tortillas
- Optional toppings: avocado slices, salsa, shredded lettuce

Instructions:

1. In a skillet, sauté onion and garlic until softened.
2. Add diced sweet potatoes and cook until tender.
3. Add black beans, chili powder, cumin, paprika, salt, and pepper. Cook for an additional 5 minutes until heated through.
4. Warm tortillas in a separate skillet or microwave.
5. Spoon sweet potato-black bean mixture onto each tortilla.
6. Top with optional toppings as desired.
7. Serve hot.

Nutrition Information (per serving):

- Calories: 280

- Protein: 10g

- Carbohydrates: 50g

- Fat: 4g

- Fiber: 12g

- Sugar: 6g

- Portion size: 2 tacos

Vegetable Paella

Ingredients:

- 1 cup Arborio rice

- 2 cups vegetable broth

- 1 onion, diced

- 2 cloves garlic, minced

- 1 bell pepper, diced

- 1 cup diced tomatoes

- 1 cup chopped vegetables (such as peas, carrots, and green beans)

- 1 teaspoon smoked paprika

- 1/2 teaspoon saffron threads (optional)

- Salt and pepper to taste

- Fresh parsley for garnish

Instructions:

1. In a large skillet, sauté onion and garlic until translucent.
2. Add Arborio rice and cook for 1-2 minutes until lightly toasted.
3. Stir in diced tomatoes, bell pepper, chopped vegetables, smoked paprika, saffron threads (if using), salt, and pepper.
4. Pour vegetable broth over the rice mixture and bring to a simmer.
5. Cover and cook for 20-25 minutes until rice is tender and liquid is absorbed.
6. Remove from heat and let sit for 5 minutes.
7. Fluff with a fork and garnish with fresh parsley before serving.

Nutrition Information (per serving):

- Calories: 250
- Protein: 6g
- Carbohydrates: 50g
- Fat: 2g
- Fiber: 6g

- Sugar: 4g
- Portion size: 1/4 of recipe

Stuffed Acorn Squash with Quinoa and Cranberries

Ingredients:

- 2 acorn squash, halved and seeds removed
- 1 cup cooked quinoa
- 1/2 cup dried cranberries
- 1/4 cup chopped pecans
- 2 tablespoons maple syrup
- 1 tablespoon olive oil
- 1 teaspoon cinnamon
- Salt and pepper to taste

Instructions:

1. Preheat oven to 375°F (190°C).
2. Brush acorn squash halves with olive oil and sprinkle with salt and pepper.
3. Place squash halves cut-side down on a baking sheet and bake for 30 minutes.

4. In a bowl, mix together cooked quinoa, dried cranberries, chopped pecans, maple syrup, olive oil, cinnamon, salt, and pepper.

5. Remove squash from the oven and fill each half with the quinoa mixture.

6. Return to the oven and bake for an additional 15-20 minutes until squash is tender and filling is heated through.

7. Serve hot.

Nutrition Information (per serving):

- Calories: 280
- Protein: 6g
- Carbohydrates: 55g
- Fat: 8g
- Fiber: 8g
- Sugar: 14g
- Portion size: 1/2 of squash (1 filled half)

Thai Peanut Noodles with Tofu

Ingredients:

- 8 oz rice noodles

- 1 block (14 oz) firm tofu, drained and cubed
- 1 bell pepper, thinly sliced
- 1 carrot, julienned
- 1 cup broccoli florets
- 2 cloves garlic, minced
- 1/4 cup peanut butter
- 2 tablespoons soy sauce
- 1 tablespoon maple syrup
- 1 tablespoon rice vinegar
- 1 teaspoon sesame oil
- Crushed peanuts and chopped cilantro for garnish

Instructions:

1. Cook rice noodles according to package instructions. Drain and set aside.
2. In a large skillet, sauté tofu until golden brown on all sides. Remove from skillet and set aside.
3. In the same skillet, sauté bell pepper, carrot, broccoli, and garlic until tender-crisp.
4. In a small bowl, whisk together peanut butter, soy sauce, maple syrup, rice vinegar, and sesame oil to make the sauce.

5. Add cooked noodles, tofu, and sauce to the skillet. Toss until everything is well coated and heated through.

6. Serve hot, garnished with crushed peanuts and chopped cilantro.

Nutrition Information (per serving):

- Calories: 380
- Protein: 18g
- Carbohydrates: 45g
- Fat: 15g
- Fiber: 6g
- Sugar: 6g
- Portion size: 1/4 of recipe

Sweet Potato and Chickpea Curry

Ingredients:

- 2 medium sweet potatoes, peeled and diced
- 1 can (15 oz) chickpeas, drained and rinsed
- 1 onion, diced
- 2 cloves garlic, minced
- 1 can (14 oz) coconut milk

- 1 cup vegetable broth
- 2 tablespoons curry powder
- 1 teaspoon turmeric
- Salt and pepper to taste
- Fresh cilantro for garnish

Instructions:

1. In a large pot, sauté onion and garlic until softened.
2. Add diced sweet potatoes, chickpeas, curry powder, turmeric, salt, and pepper. Stir to combine.
3. Pour in coconut milk and vegetable broth. Bring to a simmer and cook for 20-25 minutes until sweet potatoes are tender.
4. Serve hot, garnished with fresh cilantro.

Nutrition Information (per serving):

- Calories: 320
- Protein: 10g
- Carbohydrates: 45g
- Fat: 12g
- Fiber: 10g
- Sugar: 8g

- Portion size: 1/4 of recipe

Mushroom Risotto

Ingredients:

- 1 cup Arborio rice
- 4 cups vegetable broth
- 1 onion, diced
- 2 cloves garlic, minced
- 8 oz mushrooms, sliced
- 1/2 cup dry white wine (optional)
- 1/4 cup grated Parmesan cheese
- 2 tablespoons butter
- Salt and pepper to taste
- Fresh parsley for garnish

Instructions:

1. In a saucepan, heat vegetable broth over low heat and keep it warm.
2. In a separate large skillet, melt butter over medium heat. Add diced onion and garlic, sauté until translucent.

3. Add Arborio rice to the skillet and cook for 1-2 minutes until lightly toasted.

4. If using, pour in the white wine and stir until absorbed.

5. Add sliced mushrooms to the skillet and cook until softened.

6. Begin adding warm vegetable broth to the skillet, one ladleful at a time, stirring constantly and allowing the rice to absorb the broth before adding more.

7. Continue this process until the rice is cooked and creamy, about 20-25 minutes.

8. Stir in grated Parmesan cheese and season with salt and pepper to taste.

9. Garnish with fresh parsley before serving.

Nutrition Information (per serving):

- Calories: 300
- Protein: 8g
- Carbohydrates: 45g
- Fat: 8g
- Fiber: 4g
- Sugar: 4g
- Portion size: 1/4 of recipe

Chapter 5: Snacks and Appetizers

In this chapter, we've curated a selection of delicious and nutritious snacks and appetizers that are perfect for satisfying cravings and keeping hunger at bay. From crunchy vegetables paired with flavorful dips to savory bites and satisfying nibbles, these recipes are sure to delight your taste buds while providing the energy you need to power through your day.

Guacamole with Veggie Sticks

Ingredients:

- 2 ripe avocados
- 1 small tomato, diced
- 1/4 cup finely chopped onion
- 1 clove garlic, minced
- 1 tablespoon lime juice
- Salt and pepper to taste
- Carrot sticks, cucumber slices, bell pepper strips for dipping

Instructions:

1. Scoop the flesh of the avocados into a bowl and mash with a fork.
2. Add the diced tomato, chopped onion, minced garlic, and lime juice to the bowl. Mix until well combined.
3. Season with salt and pepper to taste.
4. Serve the guacamole with veggie sticks for dipping.

Nutrition Information (per serving):

- Calories: 120
- Protein: 2g
- Carbohydrates: 8g
- Fat: 10g
- Fiber: 5g
- Sugar: 2g
- Portion size: 1/4 cup guacamole with assorted veggie sticks

Hummus and Whole Wheat Pita Bread

Ingredients:

- 1 can (15 ounces) chickpeas, drained and rinsed
- 2 tablespoons tahini
- 2 tablespoons lemon juice
- 1 clove garlic, minced
- 2 tablespoons olive oil
- Salt and pepper to taste
- Whole wheat pita bread, cut into wedges for serving

Instructions:

1. In a food processor, combine the chickpeas, tahini, lemon juice, minced garlic, olive oil, salt, and pepper.
2. Blend until smooth, adding water as needed to achieve desired consistency.
3. Transfer the hummus to a serving bowl.
4. Serve with whole wheat pita bread wedges for dipping.

Nutrition Information (per serving):

- Calories: 150
- Protein: 5g
- Carbohydrates: 20g
- Fat: 7g
- Fiber: 5g
- Sugar: 1g
- Portion size: 1/4 cup hummus with 2 whole wheat pita bread wedges

Cucumber and Tomato Bruschetta

Ingredients:

- 2 large tomatoes, diced
- 1 cucumber, diced
- 2 tablespoons chopped fresh basil
- 1 tablespoon balsamic vinegar
- 1 tablespoon olive oil
- Salt and pepper to taste
- Whole grain baguette, sliced and toasted

Instructions:

1. In a bowl, combine the diced tomatoes, diced cucumber, chopped fresh basil, balsamic vinegar, olive oil, salt, and pepper.
2. Mix until well combined.
3. Spoon the mixture onto the toasted whole grain baguette slices.
4. Serve immediately.

Nutrition Information (per serving):

- Calories: 80
- Protein: 2g
- Carbohydrates: 10g
- Fat: 4g
- Fiber: 2g
- Sugar: 3g
- Portion size: 2 slices of bruschetta on whole grain baguette slices

Edamame with Sea Salt

Ingredients:

- 2 cups frozen edamame

- Sea salt to taste

Instructions:

1. Bring a pot of water to a boil.
2. Add the frozen edamame and cook for 3-5 minutes, or until tender.
3. Drain the edamame and transfer to a serving bowl.
4. Sprinkle with sea salt to taste.
5. Toss to coat evenly.
6. Serve warm or chilled.

Nutrition Information (per serving):

- Calories: 120
- Protein: 11g
- Carbohydrates: 9g
- Fat: 4g
- Fiber: 6g
- Sugar: 2g
- Portion size: 1 cup edamame

Roasted Chickpeas

Ingredients:

- 1 can (15 ounces) chickpeas, drained and rinsed
- 1 tablespoon olive oil
- 1 teaspoon smoked paprika
- 1/2 teaspoon garlic powder
- 1/2 teaspoon cumin
- Salt to taste

Instructions:

1. Preheat the oven to 400°F (200°C).
2. Pat the chickpeas dry with a paper towel and transfer to a baking sheet.
3. Drizzle with olive oil and sprinkle with smoked paprika, garlic powder, cumin, and salt.
4. Toss to coat evenly.
5. Spread the chickpeas in a single layer on the baking sheet.
6. Bake for 20-25 minutes, or until crispy, shaking the pan halfway through.
7. Remove from the oven and let cool slightly before serving.

Nutrition Information (per serving):

- Calories: 160
- Protein: 6g
- Carbohydrates: 22g
- Fat: 6g
- Fiber: 6g
- Sugar: 3g
- Portion size: 1/2 cup roasted chickpeas

Greek Yogurt Dip with Fresh Vegetables

Ingredients:

- 1 cup plain Greek yogurt
- 1 tablespoon chopped fresh dill
- 1 tablespoon lemon juice
- 1 clove garlic, minced
- Salt and pepper to taste
- Assorted fresh vegetables for dipping (carrot sticks, cucumber slices, bell pepper strips)

Instructions:

1. In a bowl, combine the plain Greek yogurt, chopped fresh dill, lemon juice, minced garlic, salt, and pepper.
2. Mix until well combined.
3. Transfer the dip to a serving bowl.
4. Serve with assorted fresh vegetables for dipping.

Nutrition Information (per serving):

*   Calories: 60
*   Protein: 6g
*   Carbohydrates: 4g
*   Fat: 2g
*   Fiber: 1g
*   Sugar: 3g
*   Portion size: 1/4 cup dip with assorted fresh vegetables

Stuffed Mini Bell Peppers

Ingredients:

*   12 mini bell peppers
*   1 cup low-fat cream cheese

- 1/4 cup chopped fresh chives
- 1/4 cup chopped sun-dried tomatoes
- Salt and pepper to taste

Instructions:

1. Slice the tops off the mini bell peppers and remove the seeds.
2. In a bowl, mix the low-fat cream cheese, chopped fresh chives, chopped sun-dried tomatoes, salt, and pepper until well combined.
3. Spoon the cream cheese mixture into the hollowed-out mini bell peppers.
4. Serve immediately or refrigerate until ready to serve.

Nutrition Information (per serving):

- Calories: 60
- Protein: 3g
- Carbohydrates: 4g
- Fat: 3g
- Fiber: 1g
- Sugar: 2g
- Portion size: 2 stuffed mini bell peppers

Avocado Slices on Whole Grain Crackers

Ingredients:

- 1 ripe avocado
- Whole grain crackers
- Sea salt and black pepper to taste

Instructions:

1. Slice the avocado into thin slices.
2. Arrange the avocado slices on top of whole grain crackers.
3. Sprinkle with sea salt and black pepper to taste.
4. Serve immediately.

Nutrition Information (per serving):

- Calories: 90
- Protein: 2g
- Carbohydrates: 8g
- Fat: 6g
- Fiber: 4g
- Sugar: 0g

- Portion size: 2 whole grain crackers with avocado slices

Baked Sweet Potato Fries

Ingredients:

- 2 large sweet potatoes, cut into fries
- 1 tablespoon olive oil
- 1 teaspoon paprika
- 1/2 teaspoon garlic powder
- Salt and pepper to taste

Instructions:

1. Preheat the oven to 425°F (220°C).
2. In a bowl, toss the sweet potato fries with olive oil, paprika, garlic powder, salt, and pepper until evenly coated.
3. Spread the fries in a single layer on a baking sheet lined with parchment paper.
4. Bake for 25-30 minutes, flipping halfway through, until the fries are golden and crispy.
5. Remove from the oven and serve hot.

Nutrition Information (per serving):

- Calories: 120
- Protein: 2g
- Carbohydrates: 20g
- Fat: 4g
- Fiber: 4g
- Sugar: 4g
- Portion size: 1/2 cup baked sweet potato fries

Caprese Skewers with Cherry Tomatoes and Mozzarella

Ingredients:

- Cherry tomatoes
- Fresh mozzarella balls
- Fresh basil leaves
- Balsamic glaze (optional)
- Wooden skewers

Instructions:

1. Thread a cherry tomato, a fresh mozzarella ball, and a basil leaf onto a wooden skewer.

2. Repeat until all ingredients are used.

3. Arrange the skewers on a serving platter.

4. Drizzle with balsamic glaze if desired.

5. Serve immediately.

Nutrition Information (per serving):

- Calories: 80

- Protein: 5g

- Carbohydrates: 2g

- Fat: 6g

- Fiber: 0g

- Sugar: 1g

- Portion size: 2 skewers

Kale Chips

Ingredients:

- 1 bunch kale, stems removed and torn into bite-sized pieces

- 1 tablespoon olive oil

- Salt and pepper to taste

Instructions:

1. Preheat the oven to 300°F (150°C).
2. In a large bowl, toss the kale pieces with olive oil, salt, and pepper until evenly coated.
3. Spread the kale in a single layer on a baking sheet lined with parchment paper.
4. Bake for 10-15 minutes, or until the kale is crispy but not burnt.
5. Remove from the oven and let cool slightly before serving.

Nutrition Information (per serving):

- Calories: 50
- Protein: 2g
- Carbohydrates: 5g
- Fat: 3g
- Fiber: 2g
- Sugar: 1g
- Portion size: 1 cup kale chips

Spinach and Artichoke Dip with Whole Grain Tortilla Chips

Ingredients:

- 1 cup cooked spinach, chopped
- 1 cup canned artichoke hearts, chopped
- 1 cup plain Greek yogurt
- 1/4 cup grated Parmesan cheese
- 1/4 cup shredded mozzarella cheese
- 1 clove garlic, minced
- Salt and pepper to taste
- Whole grain tortilla chips for dipping

Instructions:

1. In a bowl, combine the cooked spinach, chopped artichoke hearts, plain Greek yogurt, grated Parmesan cheese, shredded mozzarella cheese, minced garlic, salt, and pepper.
2. Mix until well combined.
3. Transfer the mixture to a baking dish.
4. Bake in a preheated oven at 350°F (175°C) for 20-25 minutes, or until bubbly and golden brown on top.
5. Serve hot with whole grain tortilla chips for dipping.

Nutrition Information (per serving):

- Calories: 90
- Protein: 6g
- Carbohydrates: 8g
- Fat: 4g
- Fiber: 2g
- Sugar: 1g
- Portion size: 1/4 cup dip with whole grain tortilla chips

Greek Yogurt Bark with Berries and Nuts

Ingredients:

- 2 cups plain Greek yogurt
- 1 tablespoon honey or maple syrup
- 1/2 cup mixed berries (such as strawberries, blueberries, raspberries)
- 1/4 cup chopped nuts (such as almonds, walnuts)
- Optional: shredded coconut, dark chocolate chips

Instructions:

1. Line a baking sheet with parchment paper.

2. In a bowl, mix the plain Greek yogurt with honey or maple syrup until well combined.

3. Spread the yogurt mixture evenly onto the prepared baking sheet.

4. Sprinkle the mixed berries, chopped nuts, and any other desired toppings over the yogurt.

5. Place the baking sheet in the freezer for 2-3 hours, or until the yogurt bark is firm.

6. Once frozen, break the bark into pieces and serve immediately.

Nutrition Information (per serving):

- Calories: 100
- Protein: 8g
- Carbohydrates: 8g
- Fat: 5g
- Fiber: 2g
- Sugar: 5g
- Portion size: 1/4 cup yogurt bark

Veggie Spring Rolls with Peanut Dipping Sauce

Ingredients:

For Spring Rolls:

* Rice paper wrappers
* Thinly sliced vegetables (such as carrots, cucumbers, bell peppers, lettuce, avocado)
* Fresh herbs (such as cilantro, mint, basil)
* Cooked vermicelli noodles (optional)

For Peanut Dipping Sauce:

* 1/4 cup peanut butter
* 2 tablespoons soy sauce
* 1 tablespoon lime juice
* 1 tablespoon honey or maple syrup
* 1 clove garlic, minced
* Water (as needed for thinning)

Instructions:

1. Prepare all the vegetables and herbs for the spring rolls.
2. Fill a shallow dish with warm water.

3. Dip a rice paper wrapper into the warm water for a few seconds until it softens.

4. Place the softened wrapper onto a clean surface.

5. Arrange a small portion of the sliced vegetables, herbs, and cooked vermicelli noodles (if using) in the center of the wrapper.

6. Fold the sides of the wrapper over the filling, then roll tightly to form a spring roll.

7. Repeat with the remaining ingredients.

8. In a small bowl, whisk together the peanut butter, soy sauce, lime juice, honey or maple syrup, and minced garlic until smooth.

9. Add water as needed to thin the sauce to desired consistency.

10. Serve the spring rolls with the peanut dipping sauce.

Nutrition Information (per serving - 2 spring rolls with dipping sauce):

- Calories: 200
- Protein: 6g
- Carbohydrates: 20g
- Fat: 10g

- Fiber: 4g

- Sugar: 6g

- Portion size: 2 spring rolls with dipping sauce

Almond Butter and Apple Slices

Ingredients:

- 2 medium apples, sliced

- 1/4 cup almond butter

- Cinnamon for sprinkling (optional)

Instructions:

1. Wash and slice the apples into thin wedges.

2. Spread almond butter onto each apple slice.

3. Sprinkle with cinnamon if desired.

4. Serve immediately.

Nutrition Information (per serving):

- Calories: 180

- Protein: 4g

- Carbohydrates: 20g

- Fat: 10g

- Fiber: 6g

- Sugar: 14g

- Portion size: 1 apple with almond butter

Chapter 6: Desserts

In this chapter, we've curated a selection of delightful treats that are not only delicious but also mindful of your blood sugar levels. From fruity delights to decadent chocolates, there's something here to satisfy every craving while keeping your health in check. So go ahead, treat yourself guilt-free with these scrumptious desserts!

Berry Crisp with Oat Topping

Ingredients:

- Mixed berries (strawberries, blueberries, raspberries)
- Rolled oats
- Almond flour
- Coconut oil
- Maple syrup
- Cinnamon

Instructions:

1. Preheat the oven to 350°F (175°C).

2. In a bowl, mix the berries with a dash of cinnamon and maple syrup.

3. In another bowl, combine rolled oats, almond flour, melted coconut oil, and maple syrup to create the crisp topping.

4. Spread the berry mixture in a baking dish and sprinkle the oat topping evenly over it.

5. Bake for 25-30 minutes, until the topping is golden brown and the berries are bubbling.

6. Serve warm, topped with a dollop of Greek yogurt if desired.

Nutrition Information:

- Calories: 200
- Protein: 4g
- Carbohydrates: 30g
- Fat: 8g
- Fiber: 5g
- Sugar: 15g
- Portion Size: 1/2 cup

Dark Chocolate Covered Strawberries

Ingredients:

- Fresh strawberries
- Dark chocolate chips

Instructions:

1. Wash and dry the strawberries thoroughly.
2. Melt the dark chocolate chips in a microwave-safe bowl in 30-second intervals, stirring in between until smooth.
3. Dip each strawberry into the melted chocolate, coating it halfway.
4. Place the chocolate-covered strawberries on a parchment-lined tray.
5. Allow the chocolate to set in the refrigerator for about 15 minutes.
6. Enjoy as a guilt-free indulgence!

Nutrition Information:

- Calories: 60
- Protein: 1g

- Carbohydrates: 10g

- Fat: 3g

- Fiber: 2g

- Sugar: 6g

- Portion Size: 3 strawberries

Frozen Yogurt Bark with Mixed Berries

Ingredients:

- Greek yogurt

- Mixed berries (strawberries, blueberries, raspberries)

- Honey (optional)

Instructions:

1. Line a baking sheet with parchment paper.

2. Spread Greek yogurt evenly on the parchment paper, about 1/4 inch thick.

3. Scatter mixed berries over the yogurt, pressing them gently into the surface.

4. Drizzle honey over the top for added sweetness if desired.

5. Place the baking sheet in the freezer for at least 2 hours, or until the yogurt is completely frozen.

6. Once frozen, break the yogurt bark into pieces and enjoy immediately.

Nutrition Information:

- Calories: 80
- Protein: 6g
- Carbohydrates: 12g
- Fat: 0g
- Fiber: 2g
- Sugar: 8g
- Portion Size: 1/4 cup

Banana Nice Cream

Ingredients:

- Ripe bananas
- Vanilla extract (optional)
- Toppings of choice (nuts, berries, dark chocolate chips)

Instructions:

1. Peel and slice ripe bananas into coins.

2. Place the banana slices in a single layer on a baking sheet lined with parchment paper.

3. Freeze the banana slices for at least 2 hours or until completely frozen.

4. Transfer the frozen banana slices to a blender or food processor.

5. Blend until smooth and creamy, adding a splash of vanilla extract if desired.

6. Serve immediately as soft-serve ice cream or transfer to a container and freeze for a firmer texture.

7. Top with your favorite toppings and enjoy!

Nutrition Information:

- Calories: 100
- Protein: 1g
- Carbohydrates: 25g
- Fat: 0g
- Fiber: 3g
- Sugar: 14g
- Portion Size: 1/2 cup

Baked Apples with Cinnamon

Ingredients:

- Apples
- Cinnamon
- Honey (optional)

Instructions:

1. Preheat the oven to 375°F (190°C).
2. Core the apples and slice them horizontally into rounds.
3. Place the apple rounds on a baking sheet lined with parchment paper.
4. Sprinkle cinnamon over the apple slices and drizzle with honey if desired.
5. Bake for 20-25 minutes, or until the apples are tender and lightly golden.
6. Serve warm as a comforting and naturally sweet dessert.

Nutrition Information:

- Calories: 90
- Protein: 1g

- Carbohydrates: 25g
- Fat: 0g
- Fiber: 5g
- Sugar: 19g
- Portion Size: 1 apple slice

Lemon Poppy Seed Muffins

Ingredients:

- Whole wheat flour
- Baking powder
- Poppy seeds
- Lemon zest
- Greek yogurt
- Eggs
- Honey
- Vanilla extract

Instructions:

1. Preheat the oven to 350°F (175°C) and line a muffin tin with liners.
2. In a large bowl, whisk together whole wheat flour, baking powder, poppy seeds, and lemon zest.

3. In another bowl, mix together Greek yogurt, eggs, honey, and vanilla extract until smooth.

4. Pour the wet ingredients into the dry ingredients and stir until just combined.

5. Divide the batter evenly among the muffin cups.

6. Bake for 18-20 minutes, or until a toothpick inserted into the center comes out clean.

7. Allow the muffins to cool before serving.

Nutrition Information:

- Calories: 120
- Protein: 5g
- Carbohydrates: 20g
- Fat: 3g
- Fiber: 2g
- Sugar: 8g
- Portion Size: 1 muffin

Chocolate Avocado Pudding

Ingredients:

- Ripe avocados
- Cocoa powder

- Honey or maple syrup
- Vanilla extract
- Almond milk

Instructions:

1. Scoop the flesh of ripe avocados into a blender or food processor.
2. Add cocoa powder, honey or maple syrup, and vanilla extract.
3. Blend until smooth, gradually adding almond milk until desired consistency is reached.
4. Transfer the pudding to serving dishes and refrigerate for at least 30 minutes before serving.
5. Garnish with fresh berries or chopped nuts if desired.

Nutrition Information:

- Calories: 150
- Protein: 3g
- Carbohydrates: 15g
- Fat: 10g
- Fiber: 7g
- Sugar: 5g
- Portion Size: 1/2 cup

Greek Yogurt Cheesecake with Berry Compote

Ingredients:

- Graham cracker crumbs
- Butter
- Greek yogurt
- Cream cheese
- Lemon juice
- Vanilla extract
- Mixed berries
- Honey

Instructions:

1. Mix graham cracker crumbs with melted butter and press into the bottom of a springform pan.
2. In a bowl, beat together Greek yogurt, cream cheese, lemon juice, and vanilla extract until smooth.
3. Pour the yogurt mixture over the crust and smooth the top with a spatula.
4. Refrigerate for at least 4 hours or until set.
5. In a saucepan, simmer mixed berries with honey until thickened.

6. Allow the berry compote to cool before spreading it over the chilled cheesecake.

7. Slice and serve with additional berries on top if desired.

Nutrition Information:

- Calories: 180
- Protein: 7g
- Carbohydrates: 20g
- Fat: 8g
- Fiber: 3g
- Sugar: 15g
- Portion Size: 1 slice

Coconut Macaroons

Ingredients:

- Shredded coconut
- Egg whites
- Honey or maple syrup
- Vanilla extract
- Salt

Instructions:

1. Preheat the oven to 325°F (160°C) and line a baking sheet with parchment paper.
2. In a bowl, mix together shredded coconut, egg whites, honey or maple syrup, vanilla extract, and a pinch of salt until well combined.
3. Use a spoon or cookie scoop to form the mixture into small mounds and place them on the prepared baking sheet.
4. Bake for 20-25 minutes, or until the macaroons are lightly golden.
5. Allow the macaroons to cool on the baking sheet before serving.

Nutrition Information:

- Calories: 70
- Protein: 1g
- Carbohydrates: 5g
- Fat: 5g
- Fiber: 1g
- Sugar: 3g
- Portion Size: 1 macaroon

Pumpkin Pie Smoothie Bowl

Ingredients:

- Pumpkin puree
- Frozen banana
- Almond milk
- Pumpkin pie spice
- Maple syrup (optional)
- Toppings of choice (granola, nuts, seeds)

Instructions:

1. In a blender, combine pumpkin puree, frozen banana, almond milk, pumpkin pie spice, and maple syrup if desired.
2. Blend until smooth and creamy, adding more almond milk if needed to reach desired consistency.
3. Pour the smoothie into a bowl and top with granola, nuts, seeds, or any other toppings of your choice.
4. Enjoy immediately with a spoon!

Nutrition Information:

- Calories: 150
- Protein: 3g

- Carbohydrates: 30g
- Fat: 3g
- Fiber: 6g
- Sugar: 15g
- Portion Size: 1 bowl

Chia Seed Jam on Whole Grain Toast

Ingredients:

- Mixed berries
- Chia seeds
- Honey or maple syrup
- Whole grain bread

Instructions:

1. In a saucepan, heat mixed berries over medium heat until they start to soften and release their juices.
2. Mash the berries with a fork or potato masher until you reach your desired consistency.
3. Stir in chia seeds and honey or maple syrup to taste.
4. Continue to cook for a few more minutes until the mixture thickens.

5. Remove from heat and let it cool completely before spreading on whole grain toast.

6. Enjoy the homemade jam on toast or as a topping for yogurt or oatmeal!

Nutrition Information:

- Calories: 60
- Protein: 1g
- Carbohydrates: 10g
- Fat: 2g
- Fiber: 3g
- Sugar: 6g
- Portion Size: 2 tablespoons

Oatmeal Raisin Cookies

Ingredients:

- Rolled oats
- Whole wheat flour
- Baking soda
- Cinnamon
- Raisins
- Coconut oil

- Maple syrup
- Vanilla extract
- Almond milk

Instructions:

1. Preheat the oven to 350°F (175°C) and line a baking sheet with parchment paper.
2. In a bowl, mix together rolled oats, whole wheat flour, baking soda, cinnamon, and raisins.
3. In another bowl, whisk together melted coconut oil, maple syrup, vanilla extract, and almond milk.
4. Pour the wet ingredients into the dry ingredients and stir until combined.
5. Drop spoonfuls of the cookie dough onto the prepared baking sheet and flatten them slightly with your hand.
6. Bake for 10-12 minutes, or until the edges are golden brown.
7. Allow the cookies to cool on the baking sheet for a few minutes before transferring them to a wire rack to cool completely.

Nutrition Information:

- Calories: 80
- Protein: 2g
- Carbohydrates: 12g
- Fat: 3g
- Fiber: 2g
- Sugar: 5g
- Portion Size: 1 cookie

Berry Parfait with Almond Granola

Ingredients:

- Mixed berries (strawberries, blueberries, raspberries)
- Greek yogurt
- Almond granola (homemade or store-bought)

Instructions:

1. Wash and dry the berries, then slice any larger fruits like strawberries.
2. In serving glasses or bowls, layer Greek yogurt, mixed berries, and almond granola.
3. Repeat the layers until the glasses are filled to your liking.

4. Top with an extra sprinkle of almond granola for added crunch.

5. Serve immediately as a nutritious and satisfying dessert or snack option.

Nutrition Information:

- Calories: 150
- Protein: 8g
- Carbohydrates: 20g
- Fat: 5g
- Fiber: 4g
- Sugar: 10g
- Portion Size: 1 cup

Mango Sorbet

Ingredients:

- Ripe mangoes
- Lime juice
- Honey or agave syrup (optional)

Instructions:

1. Peel and chop the ripe mangoes into chunks.

2. Place the mango chunks in a blender or food processor along with lime juice and sweetener if desired.

3. Blend until smooth and creamy, scraping down the sides as needed.

4. Transfer the mixture to a shallow dish and spread it out evenly.

5. Freeze for 2-3 hours, stirring occasionally to break up any ice crystals.

6. Once frozen, scoop the mango sorbet into bowls and serve immediately.

Nutrition Information:

- Calories: 100
- Protein: 1g
- Carbohydrates: 25g
- Fat: 0g
- Fiber: 3g
- Sugar: 20g
- Portion Size: 1/2 cup

Peanut Butter Energy Bites

Ingredients:

- Rolled oats
- Peanut butter
- Honey or maple syrup
- Chia seeds
- Mini chocolate chips (optional)

Instructions:

1. In a bowl, mix together rolled oats, peanut butter, honey or maple syrup, chia seeds, and mini chocolate chips if using.
2. Stir until well combined and the mixture holds together when pressed.
3. Roll the mixture into small balls using your hands.
4. Place the energy bites on a baking sheet lined with parchment paper.
5. Chill in the refrigerator for at least 30 minutes before serving.
6. Store any leftovers in an airtight container in the refrigerator for up to a week.

Nutrition Information:

- Calories: 80
- Protein: 3g
- Carbohydrates: 10g
- Fat: 4g
- Fiber: 2g
- Sugar: 5g
- Portion Size: 1 energy bite

Chapter 7: Smoothies

Smoothies are a fantastic way to pack in nutrients while enjoying a refreshing treat. Whether you need a quick breakfast on the go, a post-workout refuel, or a tasty snack, these smoothie recipes offer a delicious blend of flavors and health benefits.

Green Detox Smoothie

Ingredients:

- 1 cup spinach
- 1/2 cucumber, peeled and chopped
- 1/2 green apple, cored and chopped
- 1/2 lemon, juiced
- 1/2 inch piece of ginger, peeled
- 1 cup coconut water
- Ice cubes (optional)

Instructions:

1. Combine all ingredients in a blender.
2. Blend until smooth.

3. Serve immediately.

Nutrition Information (per serving):

- Calories: 85
- Protein: 2g
- Carbohydrates: 20g
- Fat: 0.5g
- Fiber: 4g
- Sugar: 12g
- Portion size: 1 serving

Berry Blast Smoothie

Ingredients:

- 1/2 cup mixed berries (strawberries, blueberries, raspberries)
- 1/2 banana
- 1/2 cup plain Greek yogurt
- 1/2 cup almond milk
- 1 tablespoon honey or maple syrup (optional)
- Ice cubes (optional)

Instructions:

1. Combine all ingredients in a blender.
2. Blend until smooth.
3. Serve immediately.

Nutrition Information (per serving):

- Calories: 150
- Protein: 10g
- Carbohydrates: 25g
- Fat: 1g
- Fiber: 5g
- Sugar: 18g
- Portion size: 1 serving

Tropical Turmeric Smoothie

Ingredients:

- 1/2 cup frozen mango chunks
- 1/2 cup pineapple chunks
- 1/2 banana
- 1 teaspoon turmeric powder
- 1/2 teaspoon cinnamon
- 1 cup coconut water

- Ice cubes (optional)

Instructions:

1. Combine all ingredients in a blender.
2. Blend until smooth.
3. Serve immediately.

Nutrition Information (per serving):

- Calories: 130
- Protein: 2g
- Carbohydrates: 30g
- Fat: 0.5g
- Fiber: 4g
- Sugar: 20g
- Portion size: 1 serving

Spinach and Pineapple Smoothie

Ingredients:

- 1 cup fresh spinach
- 1/2 cup frozen pineapple chunks
- 1/2 banana
- 1/2 cup unsweetened coconut milk

- 1 tablespoon chia seeds
- Ice cubes (optional)

Instructions:

1. Place all ingredients in a blender.
2. Blend until smooth.
3. Pour into a glass and enjoy!

Nutrition Information (per serving):

- Calories: 140
- Protein: 3g
- Carbohydrates: 20g
- Fat: 6g
- Fiber: 6g
- Sugar: 10g
- Portion size: 1 serving

Chocolate Peanut Butter Smoothie

Ingredients:

- 1 banana
- 2 tablespoons unsweetened cocoa powder
- 1 tablespoon natural peanut butter

- 1/2 cup plain Greek yogurt

- 1/2 cup almond milk

- Ice cubes (optional)

Instructions:

1. Combine all ingredients in a blender.

2. Blend until smooth and creamy.

3. Pour into a glass and enjoy!

Nutrition Information (per serving):

- Calories: 250

- Protein: 13g

- Carbohydrates: 30g

- Fat: 10g

- Fiber: 6g

- Sugar: 14g

- Portion size: 1 serving

Mango and Coconut Smoothie

Ingredients:

- 1/2 cup frozen mango chunks

- 1/2 banana

- 1/2 cup coconut milk

- 1/2 cup plain Greek yogurt

- 1 tablespoon shredded coconut

- Ice cubes (optional)

Instructions:

1. Combine all ingredients in a blender.

2. Blend until smooth.

3. Pour into a glass, sprinkle with shredded coconut if desired, and enjoy!

Nutrition Information (per serving):

- Calories: 220

- Protein: 9g

- Carbohydrates: 30g

- Fat: 8g

- Fiber: 4g

- Sugar: 20g

- Portion size: 1 serving

Kale and Kiwi Smoothie

Ingredients:

- 1 cup kale leaves, stems removed
- 2 kiwis, peeled and sliced
- 1/2 banana
- 1/2 cup apple juice (unsweetened)
- 1/4 cup plain Greek yogurt
- Ice cubes (optional)

Instructions:

1. Place all ingredients in a blender.
2. Blend until smooth.
3. Pour into a glass and enjoy!

Nutrition Information (per serving):

- Calories: 150
- Protein: 6g
- Carbohydrates: 35g
- Fat: 1g
- Fiber: 6g
- Sugar: 20g
- Portion size: 1 serving

Strawberry Banana Smoothie

Ingredients:

- 1 cup strawberries, hulled
- 1 banana
- 1/2 cup plain Greek yogurt
- 1/2 cup almond milk
- 1 tablespoon honey or maple syrup (optional)
- Ice cubes (optional)

Instructions:

1. Combine all ingredients in a blender.
2. Blend until smooth.
3. Pour into a glass and enjoy!

Nutrition Information (per serving):

- Calories: 160
- Protein: 8g
- Carbohydrates: 30g
- Fat: 2g
- Fiber: 5g
- Sugar: 20g
- Portion size: 1 serving

Peach and Almond Smoothie

Ingredients:

- 1 cup frozen peaches
- 1/2 banana
- 1/4 cup almonds
- 1/2 cup almond milk
- 1/4 teaspoon vanilla extract
- Ice cubes (optional)

Instructions:

1. Place all ingredients in a blender.
2. Blend until smooth.
3. Pour into a glass, garnish with sliced peaches if desired, and enjoy!

Nutrition Information (per serving):

- Calories: 200
- Protein: 7g
- Carbohydrates: 25g
- Fat: 9g
- Fiber: 5g
- Sugar: 15g
- Portion size: 1 serving

Blueberry Avocado Smoothie

Ingredients:

- 1/2 cup blueberries (fresh or frozen)
- 1/4 avocado
- 1/2 banana
- 1/2 cup spinach
- 1/2 cup almond milk
- 1 tablespoon honey or maple syrup (optional)
- Ice cubes (optional)

Instructions:

1. Combine all ingredients in a blender.
2. Blend until smooth.
3. Pour into a glass and enjoy!

Nutrition Information (per serving):

- Calories: 180
- Protein: 4g
- Carbohydrates: 30g
- Fat: 7g
- Fiber: 7g
- Sugar: 18g
- Portion size: 1 serving

Raspberry Spinach Smoothie

Ingredients:

- 1/2 cup raspberries (fresh or frozen)
- 1 cup spinach
- 1/2 banana
- 1/2 cup plain Greek yogurt
- 1/2 cup almond milk
- Ice cubes (optional)

Instructions:

1. Combine all ingredients in a blender.
2. Blend until smooth.
3. Pour into a glass and enjoy!

Nutrition Information (per serving):

- Calories: 160
- Protein: 9g
- Carbohydrates: 25g
- Fat: 2g
- Fiber: 6g
- Sugar: 15g
- Portion size: 1 serving

Apple Pie Smoothie

Ingredients:

- 1 apple, cored and chopped
- 1/2 banana
- 1/2 cup oats
- 1/2 teaspoon cinnamon
- 1/4 teaspoon nutmeg
- 1 cup almond milk
- Ice cubes (optional)

Instructions:

1. Place all ingredients in a blender.
2. Blend until smooth.
3. Pour into a glass, sprinkle with a dash of cinnamon if desired, and enjoy!

Nutrition Information (per serving):

- Calories: 220
- Protein: 6g
- Carbohydrates: 40g
- Fat: 4g
- Fiber: 7g

- Sugar: 20g

- Portion size: 1 serving

Peanut Butter Banana Smoothie

Ingredients:

- 1 banana

- 2 tablespoons natural peanut butter

- 1/2 cup plain Greek yogurt

- 1/2 cup almond milk

- 1 tablespoon honey or maple syrup (optional)

- Ice cubes (optional)

Instructions:

1. Combine all ingredients in a blender.

2. Blend until smooth and creamy.

3. Pour into a glass and enjoy!

Nutrition Information (per serving):

- Calories: 280

- Protein: 14g

- Carbohydrates: 30g

- Fat: 12g

- Fiber: 5g

- Sugar: 20g

- Portion size: 1 serving

Beet and Berry Smoothie

Ingredients:

- 1/2 cup cooked beets, chopped

- 1/2 cup mixed berries (strawberries, blueberries, raspberries)

- 1/2 banana

- 1/2 cup almond milk

- 1 tablespoon honey or maple syrup (optional)

- Ice cubes (optional)

Instructions:

1. Combine all ingredients in a blender.

2. Blend until smooth.

3. Pour into a glass and enjoy!

Nutrition Information (per serving):

- Calories: 160

- Protein: 3g

- Carbohydrates: 35g

- Fat: 1g

- Fiber: 8g

- Sugar: 25g

- Portion size: 1 serving

Vanilla Almond Protein Smoothie

Ingredients:

- 1 scoop vanilla protein powder

- 1 tablespoon almond butter

- 1/2 banana

- 1 cup unsweetened almond milk

- Ice cubes (optional)

Instructions:

1. Place all ingredients in a blender.

2. Blend until smooth.

3. Pour into a glass and enjoy!

Nutrition Information (per serving):

- Calories: 250

- Protein: 25g

- Carbohydrates: 15g
- Fat: 10g
- Fiber: 3g
- Sugar: 5g
- Portion size: 1 serving

CONCLUSION

"Vegetarian Recipes for Type 1 Diabetics" serves as not just a cookbook, but a trusted companion on the journey towards better health and well-being. Throughout this culinary adventure, we've explored the intricate dance between nutrition and managing Type 1 diabetes, discovering the boundless flavors and possibilities of vegetarian cuisine.

From the tantalizing breakfasts that greet each morning with energy and vitality to the comforting dinners that nourish both body and soul, these recipes have been crafted with care to support stable blood sugar levels without compromising on taste or satisfaction. Each dish is a celebration of wholesome ingredients, vibrant colors, and exquisite flavors, proving that eating well can be both a pleasure and a powerful form of self-care.

As we bid farewell to these pages, let us carry forth the lessons learned and the flavors savored into our daily lives. Let us embrace the diversity of plant-based foods, savoring each bite with mindfulness and gratitude. And let us remember that with knowledge, creativity, and a dash of culinary magic, we have the power to nourish ourselves in ways that promote not just physical health, but also joy, connection, and vitality.

May this book be a source of inspiration and empowerment for all those navigating the complex terrain of Type 1 diabetes, reminding us that with the right tools and a touch of culinary flair, every meal can be a delicious step towards wellness. Here's to a future filled with vibrant health, delicious food, and endless culinary adventures. Bon appétit and happy cooking!